ROAR

Feeling Defeated, Becoming Victorious

MARCELLA POWELL

CONTENTS

DEDICATION

I dedicate this book to my beautiful, smart, intelligent daughter Coriana Powell. The strength and bravery you utilize on a daily basis is beyond human. During my Cancer diagnoses you prophesied to me many times and didn't realize how much your words encouraged me to not give up. Your beautiful smile and warm touch are what keep me moving forward and knowing that I'm able to call you my best friend and daughter helps me never give up. I love you.

ACKNOWLEDGMENT

It is impossible to have completed this book without the Journey through Cancer. In writing this book, I must acknowledge those who sacrificed their time, prayers, long nights, and Early mornings to help me win the battle of Cancer. Although all glory belongs to God, I honor you for being my angels when I was in need.

Thanks to my family, friends, and loved ones. Thank you to the medical staff at The Woodland Medical Center, HCA Florida Hospital, and Baptist Medical Center. Thank you to the teachers at my daughter's school for helping her through a rough year. Thank you to my Unity Prayer family for always covering me.

Most importantly, thank you, God, for healing my body of Cancer.

INTRODUCTION

This book raises awareness of the journey of breast cancer and its impact on people's lives. The process can be a difficult one, but if we trust it, we will get through it. Life will hit us off guard, and in those moments, we must stand courageously with our heads held high. No matter how strong the wind blows. We must fight the resistance, and if we do this, we will come out on the other side. Although the journey may be difficult, we will get through it together. This book shows the strength of God in full motion.

CHAPTER 1

REFLECTION

Before 2022, I thought the extent of pain that a human could ever feel would be losing a birth parent, or should I say both birth parents. That pain felt like a sharp pain in your chest, the center of your wardrobe that left a knot and constant pressure in the same spot over time. That pain never faded away, and when a memory or voice sounded similar, something would awaken the womb so it would never go away, only be tucked away; I found out even that pain could be topped when I heard the words Ms. Powell, you have invasive cancer, and it's very aggressive. The doctor's words pierced my soul, but I was calm. No emotion: I just shook my head and nodded as if it was something else he said it seemed unreal, but it hurt. Because I could feel I knew this, indeed, was not a dream. In dreams, you don't feel pain like this. The hurt I felt, I couldn't yell or cry. I spoke in a low tone and dry voice effortlessly. I had never felt this pain before, and I knew that life just became much more accurate because I had never thought of it. At that very moment, my life flashed quickly; I began to think about all the things I still wanted to do.

I thought about who would raise my daughter if I died and if they would raise her the way I would wish. A diagnosis such as this seemed more prominent than the word spoken over my life for a moment; in all actuality, the situation seemed bigger than God for a moment only because my faith wasn't on the level to handle this type of news. I was only a babe in Christ, receiving this type of news. Don't get me wrong, I grew up in church, knew the formality, and knew scripture, but I had just surrendered my life to Jesus a few months prior. There was a saying when I was a child that when you submit your life to God, all hell breaks loose. They also said that if the devil was not messing with you, you were not that much of a threat to him. I guess both of those were true at this time in my life. I felt God hated me like he didn't love me; let's admit I was the wretch undone, the Sinner I thought of all sinners. I felt like this had happened because it was time for me to pay for the corrupt things I've done in this lifetime. With tears in my eyes, I even asked God why he hated and didn't love me; I got a reply: I'll perform it. It was not what I expected or wanted to hear, but I listened as plain as day I'll perform it.

For a brief second, I started to question my faith as a believer of Jesus, but I immediately shook the thought out of my head because I knew God was real; I had seen too many miracles I'd felt his Holy Spirit-so it was no way I was going to let the enemy use my mind that way. However, I did question why, out of all the murders, evil people, Marcella? Why did the person who I felt had been through enough, seen enough, her? Having gone through this situation, I understand now that it had to be me. We see things as happening to us, but God sees them as happening for us. His strength is made perfect in our weakness. God allows us to encounter things to restructure us to who he has destined us to become. So many times, in life, we look at situations through how we feel at the moment versus how God wants us to discern what God wants us to do and what God wants us to learn. We are human, so it's normal to take a humanistic approach, but I can attest taking a spiritual path can save a lot of stress, tears, worry, and sorrow. The humanistic approach says Oh my gosh, I have cancer; ohh my gosh, why do bad things keep happening to me? The spiritual practice says the doctor may say it's cancer, but I know healing is mine because God died on the cross over 2,000 years ago for me to be made whole.

His word says if we ask anything according to his will, he hears us, and his will is for us to prosper and be in good health. The spiritual approach says though he slay me, yet will I trust him? Weeping may endure for a night, but joy comes in the morning. This mindset assures us that we are confident in who God has made us to be and that he's in control. We can trust God at his word; even when we can't trace him, we can trust him. Trusting in God gets Rocky sometimes. Don't get me wrong; sometimes we take blows that make us lose our breath and say OK, God, OK, where are you? But keeping our hand out of it makes the storm keep passing instead of staying dormant.

The eye of the storm is the most dangerous because of the convergence at the eye-wall; the right side usually has the worst, but if we stand still, the battery will pass over. I remember we had a hurricane one year, and I lived upstairs in an apartment. I woke up in the middle of the night and didn't know what part of the storm was in, but I knew I was afraid, and the trees were hitting the windows hard. It sounded like the wind of The Wizard of Oz. I woke my daughter up, and we hopped in the car and headed to my sister's house. On the way there, a traffic light fell in front of us. We passed fallen trees on the roads and fallen power lines. We drove through high winds so strong there was a force even driving forward. We finally made it, but after making it, we realized we had gone through the eye of the storm. If we would have sat still, it would have passed over. So, I take that as a life lesson; sometimes, we must sit still and wait for the storm to pass. In the middle of the storm, we must know that it's just a storm, and this, too, shall pass. The year before the diagnosis was one of the most challenging years of my life. 2020, when the pandemic hit the world. It shook up many things mentally and emotionally, not just health-wise. It slowed me down all the way and doing that forced me to deal with things; I always overloaded myself with tasks and work. At some point, we all overwork ourselves to stop dealing with other items in our lives; we do it unintentionally. Still, our body's Natural response is fight or flight. If we aren't bravely staring down our fears and problems, we are genuinely not dealing with them. Life has taught me we will overcome the things we are willing to confront. After my mom died in 2016, I buried myself in work, whether volunteering in meetings or working.

I stayed busy every day all day, so I couldn't sit still because sitting still allowed my mind to go slow, and when it slowed down, it left a lot of space to think about my mom and that she was gone. I woke up most mornings around 5:00 a.m. I got my daughter up and ready for school. Once I sent her to school, I would either attend meetings or work. Sessions consisted of entrepreneurial endeavors or nonprofit work. I picked my daughter up, took her to play, and went home. I'd fix dinner and be in bed by 8:00 p.m. We would wake up at 5:00 a.m. and start the day again. When COVID hit, it restricted school meetings and people, and we would socially distance. So, with nowhere to go and nothing to do, I broke. My mind started thinking about Mom and never really processing her death, just living with what happened. God gave me time to deal with it. I recall looking at pictures like Why did you leave me? God, how could you let this happen? Which became overwhelming, and I found myself in a dark place. Here I am four years after my mom died, and I'm having the signs and symptoms of depression. I even replayed in my head over and over again the last day and how I could have made better choices if I knew it was the last day.

I spent that morning like this; I sat on the edge of the bed when I woke up and debated what I wanted to do. I tried to get dressed and go to the casino but second guessed if I wanted to spend time with my family first. I never knew why it was so hard to make such a simple decision that day until after that day. I chose to go to the casino, but I told my mom I was going Christmas shopping. That morning, when I entered her room, she was sitting on the side of her bed, and her head was down; she looked drained. Part of her was gone, I saw it as she existed then; I didn't know I had seen it. I was living too fast and not allowing God to guide me. I was controlling my life, which is dangerous because we should always pray that God orders our steps and will enable him to be the light on the path he leads us on. I left and went to the casino, about a 40-minute drive from the house. The drive from there wasn't long, but it was a country-long cold road with nothing but trees and deer. If you weren't looking closely, you would hit one.

After arriving at the casino, I stayed there for maybe an hour and got a phone call; it was my mom. My nephew and niece stopped up the toilet, and I yelled. I was like, why would you let them do it? How did they do it? Then I was like, OK, I'm about to head home. Ten minutes later, I called back and was like it's OK. I apologize for yelling. It's not your fault, and shortly after, I arrived home. When I reached the home, the health care nurse was there, and I remember her telling my mom she was concerned about her breathing. She wanted her to go to the hospital, but my mom didn't want to go. I remember her wanting to weigh my mom. My mom was getting up, and I said, "Stop giving her a hard time. My mom looked at me and said nobody was giving her a hard time. I'm trying to get up. I started smiling and said OK, I'm sorry. Being firm with my mother was me showing love to her. I felt I had to push her in everything she did so she wouldn't give up. Not too long after the nurse left, I convinced my mom to try to go to the hospital. Something strange was that she asked if I paid her life insurance for that month. I said yes, Mom, don't worry about any of that. I got you. I want you to get help because I love you and don't want anything to happen to you. I never thought anything of it because she always checked periodically to ensure I took care of the bills for her. My niece and nephews had just come in the night before and were also at the house with my daughter. I convinced my mom to go to the doctor. I was telling my niece to grab my mom's shoes, and I'll never forget what happened next.

I stood in the bedroom looking in the mirror and heard my mom say, Marcella.! I knew by the sound and the tone of her calling my name that she was either having a seizure or her defibrillator was going off. It happened so many times we knew what she would do or say when it was about to happen; it was that traumatizing. I looked in the mirror and said, Lord, not again; then I walked into the front. It was a process that did not go like the others this time. This process was unfamiliar; it had been over the usual length of time, and she wasn't responding to my shakes or me calling her name. She wasn't breathing anymore; I started screaming, telling the kids to go into the room and lock the door. I called the ambulance, screaming and crying.

I couldn't think of my number or address. I was crying so horribly that dispatch hung the phone in my face. I called my boyfriend and told him, then I called my Pastor, who helped me get her on the floor and told me to hold her head back. Eleven minutes seemed like two hours; the police showed up, and right after that, the ambulance showed up. My mother was DNR, meaning she's do not resuscitate, but I wanted her to live. I went against her wishes because I wasn't ready to let her go; they took her to the nearest hospital, and even though they took her, I knew she was gone because of what I witnessed with my eyes. I got the kids, and we rushed to the hospital; when they called us to go back, they told us she didn't make it. I began to weep, and in the middle of receiving this news, I heard a bunch of commotion outside the hall, and I immediately jumped up because the kids were out there. They said ma'am, don't go out there, and I screamed my kids are out there. I quickly grabbed them, and we went to a private area, and I made a phone call. I forgot my niece was a little older than the smaller kids, and she heard me mention my mom didn't make it; she started crying. My mom was like her mom because they were so close. That was one of the hardest things I have ever been through in my life, and I remember the day before all this happened, I had a heart-to-heart talk with my mom, and I told her she couldn't give up. I told her I knew she was tired, and she couldn't stop. She couldn't quit because she was a fighter, a champion. Out of all this, I remember she kept saying she wanted Christmas to be lovely, but she passed away a few days before. These years taught me to live each day like it's a last day and that the people you love come first. Also, listen to those silent things that try to guide you because that could be God's way of getting your attention. God uses anything and everything. God gets on your level every time; he understands how you think; he doesn't expect more from you than what's in you and knows what you can handle and can't handle; he created you; he knew you before you were formed in your mother's womb. He is God.

CHAPTER 2
HE CAN USE ANYTHING

After mom death, I wasn't the same; it was like her death gave me a reason to fully live and try to become everything and do everything I told her I ever wanted to do. However, it also left a big hole in my heart that is still there. What I didn't know about the spot is that you'll long for it to be filled, but no one and nothing could ever fill it. Death is something we can never escape; everyone, and I mean everyone, has to answer that call whether we are ready or not. Going through cancer taught me strength beyond all measures and how not to be afraid of it. I felt so close to death; I'd even look at my eyes in the mirror, and they would look just like my mom's eyes did when I would stare into them on her sick days. When I look at mine during those times, I didn't see life; I saw nothing. Not tomorrow, no hope, and that's how I knew something wasn't right. Luke 11:34 says the light of the body is the eye; therefore, when thine eye is single, thy whole body also is full of light, but when thy eye is evil, thy body also is full of darkness. God will show you signs and allow you to feel certain things. He will enable you to feel like something isn't right, those little things we listen to. That is God's way of talking to us, so we often look for a strong voice or a huge sign to ensure it is God. We will say, Lord, let a rock fall from the sky. But I'm learning, and in doing so, I've learned knowing God's voice is knowing that he is gentle, caring, loving, and precious. He is that small whisper that says hey, you shouldn't do that or Hey, you should go this way. God will use anything because he made everything.

I reflect on the weeks leading up to my mother's death. I still had my flowers from my father's burial, which meant the world to me because I felt like it was all I had left of him on this earth, so I cherished them and took good care of them. Suddenly, the flowers I've had for about eight years started dying. Every day, they looked sadder and sadder, withered and withered. I changed nothing and cared for them like I had cared for them for years. One day, my mom was in her rocking chair, and I was puzzled about why my plants were dying. Then I looked at my mom, looked at the plants, looked at my mom, then looked at the plants again. In my mind, I said are my plants dying because my mom is about to die.

Then I shook that thought away, but it stuck with me because two days later, I asked my boyfriend if he guessed my plants were dying because my mom was dying. He said Cella, that's a crazy way to think. Indeed, that doesn't mean that. Then, not one week later, she passed. When I called him, I was screaming I told you, I told you, she's gone. He was speechless. I said that God uses anything, anyone, and everything to get a message to his people. He gets on your level; he knows what and when you need it. Sometimes, you will feel crazy or be looked at or perceived as crazy, but during those times, you have to know without a shadow of a doubt that you know God and his voice. If God be for you, he's more than the whole world against you, so don't worry about what people say and how they look at you; choose God. That's why it's so important to know God for ourselves, not for mom, Grandma, Pastor, or dad, but for ourselves. No one soul is the same, and depending on your level of understanding and wisdom is the level God will deal with you.

In the Bible, God used a burning Bush, turned water into wine, and used anyone, especially people perceived as useless people. Don't doubt God Based on your past because your past qualified you. Yes, he's talking to you; he's showing you things; gifts are without repentance. Even if you have a past or you're not where people feel like you should be, you hold your place in God and stand on the word; he that began a good work will carry it on to completion until the day of Jesus Christ. It will be days That the only person who can get you through is God. Life will be so hard sometimes that it won't be enough, even with someone in your corner pushing you, praying, or telling you you will be OK. In those moments, you need to know God hears you and know God for yourself. Fighting cancer, I had days when I would stare off into space. People would be talking to me, but I literally would hear nothing. People told me they were praying for me, that I would be fine, that it wasn't my time to die, but those words didn't shift my emotions. All

I knew was that I had cancer, and they didn't; I felt pain; they didn't. My life was shattered. I was drowning in pain, and nobody else was; my world stopped, but everyone else world was going on. I had to talk to God and know he heard me. I had to pray and wait to hear if he was saying anything. Even when he wasn't speaking, I had to trust him enough that he would never leave me nor forsake me. There's a saying the teacher is always silent during the test, and that's true. Even when we can't hear God again, we can trust him. The safest place in the whole wide world is in the will of God, and when it comes down to trusting him, we can say with our mouth, Lord, I trust you. That's a motion. I was in that motion for months after diagnosis, and it sounded good. However, when truly trusting God, you can't fake it until you make it because God can't perform miracles with disbelief or work with disbelief. Trusting goes deeper than words. It says Lord, you made me. You know every hair on my head; you know what will happen before it happens. I wholeheartedly surrender this situation to you, and once you do that, you don't go back to it no matter what it looks like, feels like, or smells like; pray to stand on the promise of God and watch him perform it. Going through cancer, I trusted God but was trying to control everything. I was stressed out about everything; I googled everything I was afraid of. I was so afraid anytime I went to the doctor, my blood pressure would be 160 / 115. After the fourth or the fifth time, they knew they had to hurry up and Get Me Out of that room. Anxiety overtook me; when I had to get my first biopsy, my heart was pounding so hard I was afraid of the unknown. I thought I would pass out. There was a sweet lady in the room, and she was the physician's assistant performing the biopsy. and she just rubbed my arm and held my hand because she could probably see my heart beating through my chest. I didn't cast my anxieties on God or my worries; I wasn't resting in his peace. It was my battle; I was still carrying it or trying to, and it was overtaking me. The part that I didn't catch on to until later was that the word says the Lord himself goes before us; not only that, but he will be with us and never leave or forsake us. So, when I grabbed that in my spirit, it helped me realize no matter what I faced in my lifetime, if I'm facing it, I'm in God's will. He's gone before me, so he already has a way of an escape. Even when I couldn't trust the doctors, I had to trust God's word because he planned to prosper and not harm me; he plans to give me hope and a future. I've learned walking through this, God will allow situations where you have no choice but to trust him. You can't trust him off anybody else word but your own; through this, he equips us. I didn't know this several months ago; I just felt like God hated me, but who he loves, he chases. He will leave the ninety-nine sheep to find little oh you. God's love is never-ending. I remember a year and a half before my diagnosis, my daughter would have dreams and wake up crying. She would tell me Mom, I didn't want anything bad to happen to you. I'm afraid something bad is going to happen to you. I said no, nothing bad would happen to me. I told her I was fine. God had me; little did I know God was using my daughter to get my attention. The confidence I had in God was arrogant then. I felt like nothing could harm me ever. My downfall was that I felt I could have the confidence and still indulge in sin. All types of sin that weren't pleasing to God failing to realize those exact things, left the door open with the enemy. Even though God had me, God allowed the enemy to touch me. I take you back to Job in the Bible, where God asked Satan have he considered his servant, Job. Not only that, God allowed the enemy to touch his body. Sometimes, it's hard for the human mind to understand God builds us through mental, physical, or emotional warfare. He builds us by the things we say breaks us. We have to be in a place where we understand the breaking is the hand of God preparing us for greater. When my daughter told me she felt something bad would happen, I wasn't spiritually in tune with where I should have been. If I were, I would have known God was preparing me or trying to prepare me for warfare about to hit my life. But I was in my flesh and living so fast that I missed the warning signs; again, that goes back to using any and everything and everyone. God used a kid; warning always comes with big or small things; we have to be in the correct posture and position to receive and understand it when it comes. The Proverbs book confirms this by saying pride goes before destruction and a haughty spirit before it falls.

CHAPTER 3
THE BIG C

I got in the car and sat there the day I received the cancer diagnosis. I called my aunt on the phone and told her I had cancer. I was in a state of shock; I was numb. My mind was blank, and I felt the void; she couldn't believe me; she was in shock. When I hung up with her, I called my Pastor and told her she was in shock; she prayed, encouraged, and talked with me. When I finished talking to her, one of my friends located me and followed me home. When I got home, I was embraced by my aunt, my friends, and my sister. I remember sitting on the floor and staring at the bottom, still in disbelief. I was numb; people were talking, but I still don't remember everything people were telling me to this day. I remember my friends telling me God got me, but even when they told me I had to believe it within myself and not believe what they said, I had to allow God's word to come alive.

Yay, though I walk through the valley of the shadow of death, I will fear no evil. By his stripes, I'm healed. My Pastor told me to dig deep; she said I know it's hard, but you must go deep and believe. She told me to find some scriptures, read them, and quote them daily, and I did. My aunt encouraged me and told me it was done whenever I worried. She said Baby, you're already healed; it's just a process. She spoke God's word over my life and mind; she rebuked every carnal thought and imagination. She told me everyone has a process; we have to trust the process. I am 31, just hearing about a process, but my eyes and mind became open. I remember reading my Bible, and things seemed so real. I would say wow, to process it because I began processing things differently. The next day after diagnosis, I don't remember; it was so traumatic that when I say God carried me through it, he did just that. At that time, I had just started working for a company downtown, which was a great job, but with all the stress I was under, I informed them that I would not return. I went and turned in my badge, and the lady prayed with me; she encouraged me. Those sweet gestures are still remembered. The day I went to turn in my badge, my aunt, sister, and best friend wanted to ride to Foley to get my mind off the situation. We were getting gas, and I received a phone call. I answered the phone, and it was a nurse navigator from the Cancer Society. I'll never forget she got on the phone, and by her tone, I could tell she was on an assignment from the enemy. She had no sympathy, lct alone empathy; it seemed like she was trying to intimidate or scare me. She told me Ms. Powell; you have a very aggressive form of cancer. I've seen thousands of women with this type, and it spreads quickly; yours may already have spread. It would be best to see the surgeon soon because he may want you to go straight into chemo first. Then she said if it is metastatic, surgery won't work by itself, and you would have to get chemotherapy. I will never forget that moment and surely don't know how to explain what I felt other than crushed, unreal. The inside of me felt weighted, and even my heart and fear took over my body. All I knew was that I needed to live for my daughter because I didn't want anyone caring for her. I was so anxious that I couldn't drive or think, and people talking made me feel weird. Speaking made my body shake at this point; I knew I needed help from God up above. I went home, and everyone stayed with me for a while. I called my Pastor again and told her what the lady said, she said no wonder God had her praying for me that morning. At this moment, I used the scripture God watches over his word to perform it as hope that he wasn't done with me yet, and I knew he wasn't, but I felt so low and so afraid because people's comfort and presence could not take this feeling away from me that was there. Nobody could but God. Before I go forward, let me back up and tell you that If God is for you, he's more than the whole world against you. When I was diagnosed, they told me my type of cancer was very aggressive and spread quickly. The doctor tried to hurry up and get me set up with the surgery to remove it; they told me I'd get a phone call. A few weeks later, I got a phone call from the surgery center to schedule my appointment. The lady who called me was so sweet and began talking to me. While talking to me, she started declaring the word over my life prophetically, all over the phone while at work. keep in mind most jobs don't even allow you to mention Jesus. But she went all in for me, so when she didn't even know, she said Baby, it's already done. All you have to do is believe. She began to tell me of a time a woman went back for surgery and came out cancer-free. The surgeon removed all the cancer; she told me I had to believe before I went down this road. She said if I wasn't going to believe, then don't do it. I took deep breaths and said yes, ma'am; she told me I could go in next week for an appointment. She told me that the wait was at least two months. I could only thank you, Jesus, who showed God favor alone. I told her to thank you and asked her if I could have her name. She said Corinne. It took my breath away because my grandmother's name was Corinne. Out of curiosity, I asked her if she was short or tall, and she said short; I was thinking just like my grandmother. Then I asked her about her skin complexion, and she said dark brown, just like my grandmother. At this point, I had to pull over the car that I was driving, and I had to sit on the side of the road because I was so excited about how, again, God will use any and everything to show you that he's for you and that he's with you.

I was amazed at how clear God showed me he was for me, no matter what. I had to ask one last question to her to seal everything. Have you ever prayed to God and were like God? If this man is not for me, then show me. Then he shows you four times, and you still say, OK, God do one more thing to let me know, you are sure. This situation is the same, just a different scenario. I asked Ms. Corinne where she was from, and she said Greenville, AL. At this point, I knew this was a divine moment from God. It was not a coincidence my grandmother was a pastor; she was born in Greenville, AL. She was a short, dark-skinned woman, and her name was Corinne. I prayed, saying, Lord help me, Show me you're with me.

Help me believe this is your will. Looking backward now, I know it was in his will if he allowed me to go through it. So many times, the enemy will have us question God's existence in a storm or an unfamiliar place. We forget that our inability to recognize the situation does not restrain God's ability to navigate our lives. Our assignments are assigned. God has gone before us and will never leave us. Sometimes, an unfamiliar place is where God wants us precisely and needs us there to pull something greater out of us.

CHAPTER 4
TRUSTING GOD

I went into the surgery office, and as soon as I saw someone who fit the description of Corinne, I approached her and asked if I could hug her; she said yes, and I did. I filled out a packet, and I waited there with my auntie. She was beside me; we walked to the back once they called me in. They checked my blood pressure, and it was about 180 / 116. I told them I was OK; I was afraid and needed to leave their immediately. They hurried up and got me in the room. The nurse took us into the room and told me to undress from the waist up. I sat there waiting, talking to my aunt. I told her I was scared and nervous, and she said it was OK. She said God got you, baby; it's a process you got to walk through your process he got you. I put on some inspirational music to try and relax. Maybe after five minutes, the doctor came in, introduced himself, and reviewed the biopsy studies with me. He told me I was grade three invasive her two positive breast cancer; he told me it was very aggressive and said the lymph node biopsy was negative, but it could be inaccurate. He said he wanted to do a breast MRI on me, which would be the most conclusive way of knowing if the cancer had spread. I said OK, sounds like a plan. I asked him, in my case, what he recommended, a double mastectomy, and then my chances of a local recurrence would be 2%, is what he said, but he also said let's see what the MRI says. Before I left, I asked the doctor if he believed in God, and he said yes. I feel it's so important when we receive medicine or care that we pray over the doctor and the care we receive. Also, they are a God believer. After he said yes, he believed in God. I asked him if he believed in miracles and told him I was a miracle. I told him I didn't have cancer, and he laughed; I told him I had it, but God healed me from it, and I said that's why I needed the MRI to prove it. He said Well, that's what you're getting. I had to take the wheel to see God's hand move, so I was determined not to leave that place without taking the wheel. Even when he left the building, I shouted and told everyone you were about to see a miracle; now, if that wasn't taking the wheel, I had no clue what was. I called my sister. She was taking the wheel for me, too; whenever I talked to her, she would say, or should I say pscream, he did it again. She told me taking the wheel was doing the most at all times while believing in God and showing him your radical faith. At this point in my walk, no one knew what I was walking through except maybe eight people. I wasn't ashamed of what I was walking through, but I didn't feel a release from God to share it with the world. When you're under attack from the enemy, you have to fight physically, mentally, and emotionally; the last thing you need is people preying on you at your most vulnerable moment versus praying with and for you. Being on the other side of this story now, I say God forbid if I ever walk through anything similar to this again, it would probably be just me and God. The enemy will use anyone to try and make you break before your breakthrough. I learned that the enemy will come in like a flood, but God will lift up a standard. I remember a time before I got diagnosed, and God used this woman to speak to me. I was in a training class, and we were getting a facility tour. She had us all stop in front of a window, and outside of this window was a gutter; we were on the third floor of the establishment. This woman began to speak about what was in the gutter; she said when she first started working there, it was weeds and things growing in it, and one day, she noticed a flower growing in the gutter. A week later, noticing the flower growing, the gutter appeared clean, and nothing was there, but maybe a few months later, another flower similar to the first one started growing again. At that moment, I heard God speak so clearly and say even in the gutter, you can grow. I learned that no matter how dark the situation can get or how dirty you may have to get, you can grow. During the process, I held on to the fact that, no matter how much of A gutter I may seem like I'm in, I still can grow. Before I knew it, it was April eighth, the time for my first breast MRI. I never had an MRI, CAT scan, or anything; the most I've had was an X-ray at the hospital. Upon arriving, I came in contact with the staff for the MRI, and besides their name, one of the first things I asked was if they believed in God. I wanted to know before we started to make sure their lack of belief wasn't holding my miracle up because I knew I was healed, and when I got in that MRI machine, it wouldn't show up. He told me he believed in God and began to tell me about the process. During this MRI, I couldn't move, and he told me I'd wear some headphones on my ear. I also needed to do an MRI with contrast dye, so he told me they would let me know before they did it, and my body would get hot briefly when it entered my body. I got on the bed and laid down, then began to roll into the machine. About two minutes in, I heard these loud noises, and my heartbeat almost out of my chest. It was so scary, and the loud noises made it even worse. I never experienced anything like that, and the earphones were on my head, but the machine was so loud I heard through the low music they were playing. It terrified me, and honestly, that's an understatement to describe how I felt. I was so afraid. I remember my sister telling me anytime she's afraid, she quotes the 23rd Psalms, so in my head, I was saying," The Lord is my shepherd I shall not want. He maketh me to lie down in green pastures: He lead me beside the still waters. He restoreth my soul: He leadeth me in the paths of righteousness for his names sake. Yea, though I walk through the valley of the shadow of death, I will fear no evil: for thou art with me; thy rod and thy staff they comfort me. Thou preparest a table before me in the presence of mine enemies: Thou anointest my head with oil; my cup runneth over. Surely goodness and mercy shall follow me all the days of my life: and I will dwell in the house of the Lord for ever.

After my mom passed, I was placed on anxiety medicine to help cope, but I never took it until after being diagnosed with cancer. That day is a day I should have taken it and learned because, moving forward, I took it before going to any doctor's appointment. For a Breast MRI, you are laying face down on a bed, and your breasts become compressed between these machines, squeezing them tight. You can't see anything but near everything, so all I'm doing is praying, and at one point, I know the people had to hear me because they said hang in there, ma'am, we are almost finished. At that point, they began to add the contrast through the IV in my arm. My body got so hot, and it felt like I was urinating on myself, which they stated was how I would feel. At this point, it felt like I had been in there for thirty minutes, and as soon as I was about to ask for the remaining time, all the noise stopped, and they said they were complete. They told me I'd know something within five days. My nerve was so bad after that I couldn't do anything. I was shaking hard; I called my auntie and went home. I needed peace and quietness. A few days passed, and I had a phone call to go into the surgery office for results on the Monday following the call. That Sunday before the appointment, I went to church, and the preacher did an altar call and said whoever needed God to move for them right now to come to the altar. So, I ran to the altar. They anointed a small towel and prayed for me. I fell out under the anointing of God, and when I got up, I was in the spirit so heavy. The glory cloud rested in that building that day. I returned to my seat, and before I sat down, the preacher told me I was healed. She also told me it wouldn't be there when they looked again. I began to thank God for the miracle that he performed in my life, and we all began to dance and praise God. I rode with my best friend that Sunday and rested under the anointing on the way back. It was so heavy on me that I knew God had done something in me. Monday came, and me and my auntie went to the doctor's office. I was nervous a little because you know the devil must still try and make you feel defeated in a victorious battle. We were in the room, and the doctor told me the MRI said it was severe scar tissue. The scan was inconclusive. He said it was inconclusive because they found another small tumor in the machine and wanted a biopsy before it gave results. The doctor was looking at it naturally, but I was looking at it in the spirit. They scheduled me for another MRI, which was about two months away. I ended up calling the hospital and speaking with the supervisor. I informed them I needed an appointment sooner because if I had to wait two months for an MRI, I would get my breast cut off. I said that because the cancer they said I had would have spread within a month if I didn't get it out. Days had passed since I spoke with the scheduling department and got a phone call. They told me one of their machines had been down and that they were behind on MRIs but told me because I had to get an MRI-guided biopsy this time, they were trying to find a doctor who could do it. They found one to do it days later, and I was ready. The day I went in, I'll never forget my auntie was right there by my side, and she got to meet the doctor Who would be performing the biopsy. He explained the process to us very thoroughly, and before he got started, he even wanted to get another set of pictures to see if it was there. He said sometimes these things disappear, and we don't need to do anything else; nevertheless, I laid down and prayed. The machine began to take images, and after a few minutes, the bed slid out, and the doctor came in there sadly, rubbed me on the arm, and said Ms. Powell, we're going to go ahead with the biopsy. it's still there. I couldn't even reply to him; I lay silently, tears rolling down my face.I felt like my God had forgotten About me. Like he left me to die. Here I was, trusting him at his word and using my mouth to decree and declare why this tumor wasn't gone, as the scripture tells us. The scripture said if I had faith as small as a mustard seed, I could tell this mountain to move, and it would. So why was it still there? My heart ached because this tumor hadn't gone any-where. I lay there, not knowing what to expect this time; they compressed my breast with some measuring, and this time, they went through the side of my breast because they were doing an MRI-guided biopsy. They said I couldn't move one inch; if I did, it would throw off the measure-ments, and they would have to start the process all over. I said to myself I had it and would not move. They didn't tell me they used the real drill to enter the body. I was face down on the bed and heard a drill, making me panic. My mind was going a hundred miles an hour. I thought, if I pan-ic, I'm not trusting God. He didn't want me to fear. Well sud-denly I started feeling the drill, flesh jumped in then, and before I knew it, I jumped. They grabbed my arms and told me to be easy. I told them I felt every drill turn, so he gave me more numbing medicine. It worked enough for him to finish; once they got done, the doctor left, and the tech told me I'd hear something in a few days. He said usually, if it's cancer in one breast and another tumor in the same breast, then we know that cancer. Right then, I felt discouraged but didn't receive that in my spirit. I left and began to pray. I prayed that God would help me understand that his plans aren't that I perish but to prosper and be in good health. I reflected on how the devil wanted me to give up on the bi-opsy and get a mastectomy. The day I had the first biopsy, they pulled me aside and told me my insurance didn't send approval and that I had to reschedule. The way the lady said it to me was with no concern at all. It almost sound-ed like the enemy himself through her. After she told me I needed to reschedule, I said Well, ma'am, what if I can call the insurance company and get the approval. She said you have fifteen minutes; it's impossible, I said but what if I did?

Could I still get the biopsy? She said if they sent the approval over in fourteen minutes, yes. I started smiling because I knew from the look on her face that she allowed the devil to use her; I prayed for her and for time to work in my favor. I called the insurance people, and within five minutes, I had everything I needed to get the biopsy, so I knew the enemy was mad about that. Surely, God was up to something.

CHAPTER 5
MIRACLES, SIGNS, WONDERS

A week later, I found myself back in the surgeon's office waiting on results; when they came in, he told me the second tumor was not cancer and that I'd be a good candidate for a lumpectomy. I told him that was good, but I was curious about what this MRI report showed. He said to me in my case, it was wrong because it was only showing scar tissue, but he said they'd already tested the tumor and knew it was cancer. I told him or asked why the other pathology study couldn't be wrong and this be correct. I told him I didn't doubt that I had cancer, but God healed me; he said the tumor was still there. I told him the tumor was there, but the cancer was gone. I asked him a question he couldn't answer: whether an MRI machine was the most accurate way to see how cancer had spread or to read how it could not detect it in my breast. At that point, I told him I didn't want to proceed with surgery until he got another biopsy of the first tumor, and he told me ok. Two weeks passed, and the nurse called to schedule me for surgery. I said I'm not having surgery until I get the biopsy retaken. She said Well, the doctor recommends you go ahead with the surgery because the cancer is aggressive. I told her I wasn't getting surgery until I got another biopsy; at this point, I wanted to know the big deal because clearly, I felt they didn't want to give me this biopsy. The nurse said sometimes insurance doesn't want to pay for the same spot again. I told her payment wasn't an issue. If they didn't pay, I would pay out of pocket. The next day, I got a phone call from the nurse navigator, the same woman who, before I felt, was sent by the enemy; she began questioning me and tried to intimidate me. She said, what's going on? Why aren't you scheduled for surgery? Then she says why do you want another one? The biopsy, you have cancer; it's lit up on the reports. Before I knew it, I told her because it's my right as a human. I felt like God healed my body. I prayed and talked to some people I trusted, and they told me to get a second opinion and get them to do the biopsy, so I got a copy of all my files and went to get a second opinion. Tell me why I was in a place where everyone was hearing me but not listening or understanding.

I went to get a second opinion at a new facility, and this doctor called me religious. He did hear me out and listen to why I wanted a second biopsy but kept giving me the information on paper, which was cancer. He even asked me if I had kids and told me I was very young and needed to be aggressive if I wanted to see her grow up. He could tell by how I looked at him that I was not agreeing with him or that I couldn't be scared into making a decision. I knew by him Calling me religious that he didn't know God because there's a difference between knowing of God and knowing him. At this point, I felt like I had done everything I could to get them to test me again; there's a saying: stand when you've done all you can. So, after all I could do, I just cried out to God and asked, what do I do now? He replied nothing else. I have it from here; take a knee. So, I called my surgeon and told him I'd move forward with the surgery; one of my worst fears since I was a teenager was being put to sleep. It was just something in my mind that didn't regulate with being put to sleep by man when God made me. I had a hard time trusting someone else to put me to sleep. I figured when God wanted me to sleep, he'd allow me to rest at night. It did not sit right with me even though God made the men, and they went to school for everything they did. I didn't want anyone controlling me in my awareness. The way I felt, if God wanted me to sleep, he'd allowed me to rest. On the morning of surgery, my aunt and I met downstairs and checked in downstairs. Anxiety overtook me, and the more I prayed, the more anxious I became. I tried to quote scripture but wasn't calm enough to even receive the word. Filling out the paperwork in the lobby was so overwhelming because here I was, just turned thirty two years old with cancer. My mind reflected on when I was younger, and my mom would be in the hospital filling out the same paperwork. My prayer from when my daughter was born was, Lord, allow my daughter to have a healthy mom, allow her to have a mom when she's old, allow her kids to have grandparents. These were things that troubled my heart. After all, we learned the hospital from the bottom floor to the top floor because our parents were always sick, and having to fill the paperwork out took me back to that place mentally. When I finished the paperwork, I had to go upstairs to pre-op. My aunt began to encourage me and rubbed my back, reminding me that this process would pass over. As we were getting up, one of my best friends at the time hugged me. We began to go upstairs; we had to dial A number on the phone to proceed. My hands were sweating, and I was breathing deeply. the door opened to the lobby, and they said Ms. Powell. My aunt told my best friend that she could go to the back first since she had the kids and would come back next. We got to the back room, and the nurses told me I needed to urinate and change clothes. I remember being so afraid I couldn't move; I just needed a minute. After taking deep breaths, I went and used the restroom and changed clothes. I came out and laid on the bed; I felt numb because I trusted God and thought it wouldn't go this way. I wanted it to go my way, I wanted my mom, I wanted to cry, I wanted to throw a tantrum and leave. My friend could tell I was worried, so she called her mom, who was my Pastor, and she prayed with me. Shortly after, the nurse came in and tried to give me some medicine. I told her I had to use the restroom, and I got the phone from my friend and went to the bathroom. The Pastor was still on the phone, and she began talking to me. I just started crying, and I did not want to go through this at all. I was on the edge of a mental breakdown, it felt like. Through all of that, the devil didn't want me to know that I was on the verge of a breakthrough. I learned he's a lying wonder, and I've also learned he will cause the most worry and frustration about situations that God already has worked out. The weapons will form, but the Bible says no weapon formed will prosper. So, to use the word formed in an aftermath means it's already formed. That means when God created you and me, there were assigned weapons with our name on them that would come our way, but it also says it won't prosper. So, no matter how big or small the situation may be, God has already worked it out. The Pastor prayed, and after being in the restroom for about twenty minutes, I finally came out. When I came out, my friend hugged me and told them I would take the medicine by the time she was leaving. My sister came in, and of course, she could sense the anxiety and just flat out told the people in charge to give me some strong medicine. She laughed at me because I was so quiet when they gave me the medicine five minutes later; it worked, but I didn't want to take it. At this moment, I reflect on times in my life when God was the answer, but I chose to go my own way; mature me now know that God is an absolute gentleman and never forces his way onto anyone, but he stands constantly knocking saying if we trust him, he can move the mountain that is impossible to move. He can and will get in the valley with us if we trust him. We won't have to fear evil because he's always with us. I remember going to the back, and my aunt Wanda came back; she hugged me and said, "Baby, you're going to be just fine. I was so nervous because I had only had one other surgery. As they began rolling me back, I quoted the twenty third Psalm again in my head, giving me peace. When I got to the room, it was a bright light, and maybe six or seven people were there; they asked me to get on the other table and gave me a mask. I breathed into it a few times, and the next thing I knew, I was waking up being rolled in post-op. I looked around and couldn't believe it was over. It seemed as if I had just gone to sleep. I asked if my aunt could return, and they said yes. I still was sad, but I began to tell God thank you because he kept me. I was so afraid, and now I was feeling like for what? God takes care of his own. Walking out of that showed me that all the fear, frustration, and anxiety I felt in the prior moments was just a distraction from the enemy. I should have kept my eyes on Jesus, and now I knew that, but again, I am human, so I didn't beat myself up. I remember my aunt coming back, asking me if I was OK, and helping me get dressed. The nurse I had that day talked to us and told us his wife had gone through cancer a few years ago. I knew the Lord was showing us each day that we can get through this if we trust him. I remember being pushed down in the wheelchair and put in my aunt's car; from that to making it home, I'm not sure what happened because the medicine made me sleepy. My aunt helped me out of the car into the house, and I rested. Nothing can compare to the fear I had that day in my life. The feeling was an experience that felt so unreal, but I can say today I've never seen the righteous forsake me. I was in pain over the next few days, and finally being able to get up, I removed the gauze to look at the surgical sites I was cut underneath my right breast and at the top of my right armpit to look at the surgical site, and it made me emotional. Still, it helps me remember where God had brought me from. Healing took place slowly; during that time, I wondered if the scar would fade or if it would be there. Today, none of that even matters; what matters is that the love of God brought me through one of the roughest battles of my life. At a time when I didn't know if I'd smile again, he kept me. When the devil came in like a flood, God lifted a standard. Sometimes, I would look at myself in the mirror in disbelief and say, " Wow, you have cancer. I was in shock for the longest; I couldn't believe it. Right after my diagnosis, like a week or two, my uncle died of cancer. It was so discouraging to me initially because the devil put in my head, you're going to die just like him; you're next. Having that in the back of my head but trying to fight the negative things and keep moving forward was hard. I had to develop confidence within myself and God that healing was mine. It was so easy for people to tell me to trust God When they weren't the ones walking in my shoes; they weren't the ones diagnosed with cancer. I was trusting God, but I still had to walk through it. When I developed the confidence within myself and with God that healing is mine, I started putting crazy faith and crazy praises on it and the victory in this situation. I even remember going to my uncle's funeral, and the Holy Spirit rested on me so strongly that the day of mourning turned into a victory for me. I began to praise God; I ran all over that church. People probably thought I was crazy because I was doing all this at a funeral. Everyone was so sad, and I was too because my uncle was such a sweet man, and I loved him forever, but God showed me that I still have life and was grateful for life here. My uncle was laid out in the casket dead, showing me where I could be, but the grace of God allowed salvation. So, all I knew was how dare I not send a declaration of praise to heaven, thanking God for what he has done for me. After that day, I told myself to stay focused on God, and to get through it, I had to sacrifice my time, my day, and what I did. I cut communication almost with everyone because I was in a place, but God was trying to get me emotionally somewhere else. I started praying more and seeking God for a deeper relationship with him. I knew to get through this, I needed all the voices in my head to stop. well, let me say the enemy knows when you're on the right track, and he's going to throw everything to get you to ensure you don't get there.

CHAPTER 6
THE PROCESS

Two weeks had passed since my surgery, and it was time to follow up. It was a Monday, and I was excited to get the great report. I went into the office, sat down, and waited about twenty minutes before the doctor came in. He immediately told me he had good and bad news, and I started shaking and asking if it was a prank. I told him to give me the bad news, and he said they didn't get clear margins and needed to go back in immediately. I felt anger, rage, hurt, and frustration. My exact words were What do you mean, why! He said about 15% of the time, we have to go back in to get clear margins because we cannot get them. I told him that was bull crap and asked why he didn't get everything the first time. I said Well, what's the good news? He said I had something called DCIS, and it's the beginning stages of cancer, and they can get that before it transforms into cancer. At that point, I was angry and tired of statistics and percentages because I seemed to be in the unlikely percent. I left immediately, turned off my phone, and drove around crying and screaming, asking God why he kept allowing these things to happen to me. I felt I shouldn't have to go through all those battles. I felt like he gave me to the wolves; it was so much for me to process, and even though people knew God would bring me out, I knew I still had to go through it. I felt I was at my Max; I felt like I couldn't take any more. I just wanted to cry and scream at home, but I had to gather myself and smile because I still hadn't told my eight-year-old that her mom had cancer. Writing this chapter, I begin even to weep because thinking about the pain, I felt pain even on the other side. It brings my emotions into play. So, for those of you who are reading this and are currently fighting for your life, and it seems like it can't get any worse, or you will never make it out of the storm, I know how you feel. I understand. I know how it feels to cry yourself to sleep and sit in a room where everyone is moving, and you're in your world. I know how it feels to feel like everyone in the room is moving and you're stuck still, and I know how it feels to be so stressed that you have no appetite. Amid that, please also know you must trust God when you can't trace him, and he will allow you to smile again, breathe again, and have joy again. Even at our lowest, he will reach down and lift a standard; he will lift you even if he has to reach way down. If we skipped the process, we wouldn't be who God intended for us. The process we think, and the process God has for us are different, but if we trust God in his word, he will never put us to shame. After that appointment, I wasn't OK, but I had to trust God. I had no choice but to wait for my next surgery.Between those appointments and my surgery date, I remember one night my excision came open; I was so afraid, so my friend came and picked me up. Her mom was on the phone with me, and I just started panicking because blood was pouring out of my breast. She told me it was fluid and happens after the surgery sometimes. All the blood had come out when I got to the hospital. I was happy but shaken up because it added one more thing to a list of already long things. Days had passed, and Before I knew it, time passed, and it was time for surgery again. I was a little more comfortable because the staff knew me, and I knew them. I wasn't as afraid to take the medicine or to do the surgery because God had proven to me that his hand was on my life. Once again, I was in the back awaiting surgery, and my aunt was with me. We prayed as they began pushing me in the back, and then I prayed the twenty third Psalm; it gave me peace once again. Once I was back there, they began reading the procedure and standard protocol; I started dozing off again. I woke up, and before I knew it, surgery was over. I was so thankful and ready to go at the same time. Surgery this go around was a little more painful, which I expected because they returned to the same spot. I just had surgery, and previously, the doctor told me if they didn't get everything this time, they would go ahead and do a double mastectomy. I remember people were like go ahead and get them cut off now. Before cancer, I would have, but it's different and more difficult when you have to decide on your health. Also, just reading the information, I learned that removing the breast didn't stop the cancer from returning; it only stopped local recurrence. It could still come back in other parts of one's body, which is metastatic. I wasn't worried about that and still am not worried because God healed me, so it would never return. That's what I stand on every day; I decree it would never touch me nor my bloodline again, and because God is the greatest power, we can decree a thing, and it shall be established. I know it's already done, and that's the confidence we must have in Jesus Christ. Fast forwarding to the doctor's follow-up, I went in that day and told God I wouldn't let him go until he blessed me. I prayed and told God I wasn't leaving that place until these people gave me good news. I believe God knew what I meant, and I meant it from the bottom of my heart because when I went as the doctor walked in, I was like, can you give me the bad news first?He looked puzzled; he was like there was no bad news. he said we got everything, and my aunt started rejoicing. I asked him if he was sure because I didn't want it to be a temporary happiness. I was so glad, and I just was afraid that it was a temporary joy. He told me they got all of the tumors out, and he also said it was good that they went back in because half the tumor was still inside of me. He told me he was referring me to an oncologist for radiation and maybe a chemo pill. I didn't understand why I needed either when the cancer was gone. He then began to go over the recurrence percentage, and I told him it wasn't coming back. I learned as a believer it's important to stop the enemy in his tracks, especially regarding your life and health. No matter if it's the doctor, a judge, or whoever, never allow them to speak about anything negative in your life. Speaking about your life doesn't have to be directly mentioned; it can be a certain situation or a general conversation. The moment it's spoken in the atmosphere, we have to take it down in the spirit; we do this by openly declaring the opposite and decreeing the word of the Lord. Even when we fear or when fear sits in and doesn't want us to do it, we say God has not given us the spirit of fear but of love, joy, and a sound mind. We are blessed; everything we touch is blessed, and everything we say is blessed. We move mountains when we know this and walk in confidence and authority. God has confidence in us, but the real question I've learned is do we have confidence in him. Surgery was over for now, and a few weeks later, I found myself stepping into the oncologist's office. The day I went, I had my auntie and my giddy with me. Honestly, I felt blessed because I knew without a doubt if no one else was going to war for me in the flesh, these two were. I was nervous and anxious, something God tells us not to be, and no matter how much I tried to relax, I couldn't. I believe that day; my blood pressure was one hundred ninety over one hundred ten. They asked me if I was OK if my head was hurting.I told them it was anxiety and I needed to hurry up and leave. Not long after I met the oncologist, he went over my profile with me and the medical, and then he told me the plan he felt was best. He recommended two types of chemotherapy and follow-up with Herceptin and immunotherapy for a year. The doctor said since the cancer was aggressive, he needed to be as aggressive as possible, especially since I was young and had no prior sickness. I was upset because I thought I would be a candidate for a pill treatment or chemo and not have to do the rough stuff. He told me since I was young, I needed the aggressive stuff. They needed to be as aggressive as possible; with all honesty, I felt like I was being lied to and didn't know what to believe. I felt like I was being lied to because we always hear that cancer is one trillion-dollar industry, and I honestly felt like I was going through things that I didn't necessarily have to do. If I didn't know anything else, I knew the tumor that had cancer was gone, and I knew it didn't spread. Even with him reading my pathology report, I felt that was confirmation. I say that because when diagnosed earlier, they told me it was stage 3, and my oncologist told me it was stage 1. Not even a full centimeter tumor when he said that; I rejoiced and thanked God. I knew then that God had gotten in the middle and changed things for me. When they first started, the tumor seemed larger and spread to my lymph node, so it went from being spread to my lymph node basically two controlled and smaller. That still didn't change the fact that I had to do chemo, and I was sad; he told me if I didn't, my cancer would be back in just a matter of time. He said I felt good at the moment, but two or three years down the road, maybe it would be back, or maybe it'll be back in six or seven years, but he felt it would be back. He recommended doxorubicin and taxol. Besides chemo, he told me I needed surgery to get a port placed in and radiation. The port was a medical device placed in the left artery to get the chemo through. At this point, I was overwhelmed; I needed chemo and a different surgery. Everything was moving so fast I didn't even feel like I could breathe or get a breath in. The oncologist did break it down to me to help me understand why I had to put my body through this, which was really to make sure the cancer was gone and to lower the risk of coming back. The doxorubicin, also known as AC red devil chemo, is supposed to kill cancer cells anywhere in the body. The taxol is supposed to be more targeted for breast cancer, and they say it kills the cells that AC chemo left behind. Watching videos of people battling cancer and going through the same thing would help prepare me, but boy, was I wrong. After leaving that day, they scheduled me for surgery to get a port. I was scheduled for a chemo Class a day before surgery and for chemo the day after surgery. I even asked if I could start that soon after surgery because I felt it was going too fast. I needed a break; I needed them to slow down and understand what I was going through and feeling. The doctor told me he had people get the port that morning and start chemo that afternoon. I guess there was no way to get out of that. The surgery date for the port came, and in no time, so did the chemo class. At the chemo class, they reviewed the drugs they would be giving me and the possible side effects of the medicine. The doctor I had was heaven-sent; she took her time with me, and she made me feel like I was human. She listened to me; she sat there and understood how I felt with anxiety and fear. She let me know that I could get through it. When she spoke to me, I knew God was with her because she had a gentle and peaceful spirit, and I will never forget her. I had a hard time meeting new nurses or, should I say, encountering them and trusting what they said. For example, here I am, never met them a day in my life, and they are telling me that I will give you this medicine that's almost to kill you, but you won't die. I want you to trust me to give it to you. I was so afraid it was so hard for me, but her spirit connected, and I knew that God was showing me that it was OK to move forward. My giddy also reminded me that faith was not in man from the beginning but God. I learned that if our faith is in men, they will always let us down; that's something we can bank on. But if we put our hope and trust in Jesus, we will be OK. I was still nervous, but I was able to move forward. I had to depend on God; I had to rely on Him, and speaking from this moment in my life, he's never let me down. Now, I pause here and say battling cancer is not just battling cancer; battling cancer is adjusting to the new you. Battling cancer warfare, spiritual warfare, battling losing friends, battling letting go of friends because they don't understand the new you and that you're not the same person because cancer does change who you are. It changes how you think and act, and keeping your mind strong enough to mentally coach yourself into not giving up on life is a whole job. There were days I had to coach myself to fight mentally, and sometimes, on these days, I'd have to explain to people in my life that was closest to me why I hadn't called them, why I was acting different, or why I was quiet. Later I realized I didn't no longer have to do that.

CHAPTER 7
LAW OF CANCER

The day of chemo was two days before the start of school. Giddy and my Pastor at that time came over. I had so many emotions I was scared out of my mind and didn't know what to think, but honestly, I felt God would rescue me. I just knew he was.

In my head, I thought any minute they would say the biopsy results came back and it wasn't cancer or that I wouldn't have to go through the process, remember that word. I just knew God was about to stop the sun and fix everything. I could finally awaken from the horrible dream. Well, it didn't work out like that. After labs, I quickly found myself in a private suite taking anxiety medicine, which is the protocol to relax you before chemo; the nurse came in and introduced herself and told me since it was my first time, they would be going extremely slow in case I experienced any side effects or medical issues to the foreign substance. I had two different premeds than chemotherapy. The first medicine was about forty five minutes in IV format, placed through my port. The second medicine was about an hour and a half, and the chemo was about two and a half hours. I remember feeling flushed with one of the pre-meds and receiving the doxorubicin, also called the red devil. The color of the meds was red, and it was a bright red. Even now, the thought of it makes me sick to my stomach. I remember getting hooked up to it and following the medicine with my eyes through the tubes. As it began to get closer to my veins, I started panicking, and Pastor kept telling me a story of trying to keep my mind off of it. Still, to this day, I couldn't tell you what the story was about; my Pastor intended to keep me from looking at the medicine with the meds in my body. I was disappointed and shocked because my faith said God would stop it. He would intervene; however, that was not the Lord's plan. I couldn't believe I was getting chemo. At that moment, everything began getting so real to me, and I took a deep breath, exhaled, and just bathed in the fact that I had cancer. So, my question is, what do we do when God doesn't answer us according to our wants or desires? Do we still trust him? Yes, because it's his will, not ours; he knows his plans for us. When God doesn't answer, we stay, stand, pray, and know he is God. Chemo felt weird going in my body, but I think at that very moment, it was more of a mental thing as I sat there in disbelief. The more I got the medicine, the more I felt out of it; in a sense, I felt like someone was clogging me up with the glue. I felt heavy inside, and surprisingly, I could leave and walk out. They told me in three or four days, I would feel sick like a car hit me, and I would feel that way for a few days, and then it'd just go away all of a sudden like nothing ever happened. Well, as soon as I got home that day and walked inside, I fell on my couch. By the time I got home, I had no energy. I remember giddy coming in to use the restroom, but I could not physically move; I just lay there. She locked the door when she left. I felt so bad, and this weird feeling was in my stomach. It felt like I was nauseous, but in the middle of it, it felt like I had a hole in it. I believe I stayed on the couch for a few hours, and when I got up, it was only to go to bed. The next morning, I woke up, and I began feeling better. I went to get my niece to drive me around to do some last-minute things for my daughter before she had to go to school. Around lunchtime, I started feeling bad, and the feeling started coming over me quickly, so I stopped at Firehouse Subs to see if that would make me feel better. After that, I went to my friend's house, and as soon as I got there, I felt like I needed to lie down and rest. I went upstairs to her house and laid down, and when I did, it felt like everything fell on me at once. The best way to describe what I felt was abnormal. I was severely nauseous and hot and felt run over by a car. I was beyond speechless when people talked to me; I couldn't even respond; I responded by humming. Hours passed, and I didn't feel the strength to get up. The more I lay there, the more paralyzed I became. It came on so strong and quick that I was speechless. I wasn't even able to go home. I had to stay there, and my friend's husband took my niece home. My friend went to my house to get my daughter's school stuff, and we had to stay there for a few days. As bad as I felt they didn't let me leave, I couldn't leave due to how sick I was. Every day was a blur, and I only remember snaps of the day. I remember waking up the next day and being so weak all I could do was watch my daughter leave for her first day of school. I felt so bad I felt clogged up and like I was dying. I know I haven't died before, but if I had to describe it, I would say it felt that bad. I heard talking while lying down, but it hurt to even open my eyelids. When it was time to get up and go to the restroom, I would take everything I had, get up, and try to make it. I didn't eat the first two days; all I did was lay in the same spot throughout the day. I would wake up, but it was literally to open my eyes. I found myself going back to sleep. Chemo was the hardest thing in my life I went through. To describe it would be awake but lifeless. My body felt so weighted down that I remember waking up in the middle of the night and praying to God to help me. One day felt as if it was five days. Around the third day, I could sit in bed and eat frozen grapes. Even now, I pray God bless my friend and her husband for allowing me to stay there those days following my first chemo. Every morning, I heard her husband praying in his prayer closet; it helped to hear him pray because I couldn't even pray for myself then. When I was even able to get up, I started dialing in on the prayer line I used daily; it's called Unity Prayer. the phone number is 267-807-9601, and the access code is 519924; it begins at 5:30 a.m. Central Standard Time Monday through Saturday. I felt like the chemo got me to the place where I could barely hold on any longer, and then I got relief when I got to the point where I'd say I couldn't do it. Then God gave me a remarkable strength, and I felt relief from the chemo. I feel what helped me keep going was knowing God went through so much worse for me and that he was with me. Years ago, chemo was the most horrible thing of all time, and it is, don't get me wrong, but I've come to find out that with so many new diagnoses over the years. Drugs for side effects have become stronger on the market, which helps us with many symptoms and side effects. Before I knew it, it was Saturday. That's the day I felt seventy five percent back to myself; when I woke up that morning, it felt so weird because I was expecting the horrible feeling, but in a sense, I felt normal, just weak. That day, I just laid around and ate lunch with the kids, then went home with my daughter. We hadn't been home in three days, and I was so excited to be home, to feel better. I was so happy to be able to comfort my daughter and myself that I was dreading the next treatment. I only had one week before it was time to do chemo again.

As much as I tried to prepare for this treatment again, I couldn't. The week went by so quickly that I didn't know what to do. Before this treatment, I decided to tell my eight year-old daughter about the diagnosis. I asked a few people what to do and how to tell her. some said don't tell her, but my daughter was smart, and this time, she started asking why they would make me sicker every time I went to the doctor. It was heartbreaking, so I sat her down on a Friday night and told her I was sick. The next words that came out of my mouth changed her life forever. I told her I had cancer, and she started shaking badly, crying, crying, crying, hyper-ventilating, and all I could do was hold her and fight back tears. She said no, mom, not cancer, not cancer mom. I just kept holding her. I then told her to breathe; she was so trau-matized I thought she would pass out. I then began to tell her that the cancer was gone and that only a little bit was in me. I got a piece of paper and drew three different size circles. One being a small circle, one being a big circle, and one being a medium circle. Then I asked her I said sweetie, out of those three spots on the paper, which size do you think the cancer was, she said the big circle. I told her no. I told her my cancer was small, like the dot, but it's gone now. Then I told her they cut it out of me and showed her my scars, which probably wasn't a good idea because she started to freak out, but I wanted her to know what I was going through and that I was going to be OK, we were going to be OK. At that moment, I turned into Wonder Woman. I embraced my baby so tight until those tears stopped and until she believed every word I said. I even told her I still had to get medicine that would make me sick but explained to her that it was getting all of the small cancerous cells out of my body, if it's any left. I also told her that God needed to use a body in the earth's rim to get glory, and I told her he chose mine to use, so I had no choice. But I assured her God controlled this situation; that weekend was one of the most memorable. I spent most of the days cuddled up with my daughter. That Sunday was here, which meant the next day was treatment. I told my friend I was staying home for this treatment. I spoke with Giddy and my aunt, and they were willing to get my daughter from school for me and stay with me for the first few days after treatment, so it was time. Here I was on the day of treatment. Giddy took me, and it was a process. I didn't want to be there because I knew what was coming. When we got labs done and checked with the nurse, she said it wouldn't improve. It would get worse, but I would get through it. That was not the encouragement I wanted to hear. Treatment was usually three to four hours. It felt great having someone you love beside you during the process. Giddy was right there, and even with her there, I texted my auntie and other people just because I wanted to keep my mind off everything happening. By the end of treatment, I felt exhausted, like a weight was pushing my physical body down to the ground. I got up and walked downstairs after treatment. Giddy would pull the vehicle up, and I would get in and lay on her shoulder. When we got home, my aunt Veronica was home with my daughter, and I just went straight to bed. Laying in bed, I could hear them doing homework with her, but my body slowly was shutting down. The chemo was feeling all the parts of my body, and I didn't have much strength. I was tired in my head; I felt like God had forsaken me each time I got the chemo. It made me feel so horrible, and now and then, it still was hard to believe poison was going into my body. This round was horrible more difficult, and the medicine affected me worse. I threw up more, couldn't eat or drink, and moaned most of the time. My body hurt, and I was in so much pain. The next day, I'd have to get a shot in my legs to bring up my white blood cells, which made my body ache more. After a few days, I was still sick, and Giddy took me to see the oncologist. They had to start giving me fluids in the IV so it could hydrate me. A few days later, I started feeling a little better and getting my strength. It was a roller coaster: one week up, next week down, one week up, next week down, one week up, the next week chemo. The chemo began to affect me so badly that I had to get my next dose lowered and IV fluids for the next three days after treatment. On my weakest days, I tried to remember prayer was the most powerful thing. Prayer is power more powerful than chemo.I had to keep saying that I had to keep saying and reassuring that God had me, that he'll never leave or forsake me, that there was power in the blood of Jesus. The four AC chemo were brutal to my body, mind, and spirit. To describe it would be purposely shortening the details in this chapter and of the third and fourth dosage because of how painful it is to relive it in my mind. But after four chemos that I felt would destroy me and what I couldn't see myself overcoming, I finally found myself on the other side of that one.I would say it was the hardest thing I've ever done.

CHAPTER 8
THE BLOOD OF JESUS

Before I knew it, it was time for Phase Two. I was completely bald; eyelashes and eyebrows were gone. Any hair on my body was gone; my body had a few weeks of recovery from the previous chemo. The symptoms I was experiencing had lightened up, and I wasn't vomiting; I was excited to feel better. The doctor let me know this go around would be a lot easier on the body. Even though it was still chemotherapy, it would be more tolerable. I tried to convince the doctors numerous times that I no longer needed the medicine. I was letting them know God did it for me, so I didn't have to continue, but they insisted I continue treatment. This new Phase I was getting was for twelve rounds, and I was also getting immune therapy to slow the reproduction of the Her two gene in my breast. Every week, I was at the doctor receiving the treatment, and by then, I started seeing a cardiologist because of the chemo and

Herceptin, which is all toxic to the heart. I began receiving echocardiograms every three months, and the first time I got one, my strain levels were down, and I was so discouraged afterward. Can I be honest.? I was like, God, I trusted you, and you let this medicine hurt my body. I was an emotional wreck for about twenty minutes, and the Holy Spirit knocked me on the head.

Scriptures started falling in my heart, and I started saying life and death are in my tongue's power. By God's stripes, I'm healed, so I'm already healed. Though it slays me, will I trust him? After crying and quoting the word, I developed a new stance with the situation I decreed daily. I prayed over my heart and the strain level every day and stood on the word of God that the treatment would not damage nor affect my body. When I returned for the subsequent echocardiogram, the strain level was back up; for the duration of therapy, I would receive echocardiograms every three months. I also would follow a cardiologist for life, and I honestly was OK with that because my mom passed of congestive heart failure, so having a heart doctor was in the future for me. I was fighting in the middle of a storm, but the storm, indeed, was passing over. There were days when I thought or reflected too much, and it began to shake me. I remembered and thought, wow, you have been through a lot. Then I heard the Holy Spirit say that thinking about the hurt will consume us. If we think about the pain that consumes us, look to Jesus.

A new year, and finally, I was done with chemo and at a consultation with the radiologist. I was relieved and happy that God was finally answering my prayers. He was coming through for me. At my talk, I was a bit disappointed because I thought I would only need targeted treatment, meaning I would only need radiation to a small part of my breast. Still, the recommendation per type of cancer I was diagnosed with was the whole breast. I was upset because I felt that I was over-treatment but blessed. After all, it wasn't an option for so many. I prayed a day or two and told them we could proceed with the plan. A few days before treatment, I went into pre-op; for this process, they laid me down, got a permanent marker and some plastic tape, and laid me on a table with no cushion.

There were two giant machines, one in the back of me standing upright and one directly over me. They began to take scans of the breasts and the front of the tumor markers, marking over my breast and again on every area, even on my side. For every X they drew, they also put a piece of tape over it to help keep it on. Once they completed that, they provided me with my schedule, and I started radiation promptly. On my first day, I wasn't nervous. I had peace, so I knew God was with me. After radiation, I was fatigued; the process was quick. For about three to five minutes, I felt nothing while it was going on. The machines' noise frightened me the first time, but I was at peace.

The first few days were fine; it wasn't until the 6th day that I started feeling new symptoms. My right side was very sore to touch, and my breast was highly uncomfortable. I had to stop wearing a bra because the pain was unbearable. Over the next week, I felt more tired and sluggish and sluggish. I was moving, but it took so much energy out of me that by day twelve, I was weak. The radiation site became so burnt that I had to get prescription cream to treat it because nothing over the counter was helping. Under my breast began to blister a little, and how bad it felt, I was surprised it didn't look worse. At that moment, twenty-eight days later, I was weak but ringing the bell. Yet again, I didn't know the most challenging part wasn't over for me yet. Every day after that the pain grew more intense. I even called the doctor to ask him why I was burning and hurting worse than I was while I was in treatment. Water irritated it. I couldn't lay on my right side at all or wear a bra, and even after two weeks of no radiation, it was still burning. My skin started peeling, and the peel kept going under my breast and armpit; all my skin started peeling off, and under my breast, my skin changed to another color. Third-degree burns were present under my breast; I remember being so worried and calling the doctor, telling them to get me in, only to say that that's regular radiation burns. That's all they could do, as dry as it sounds, because it was a process. The process again brought my mind back to trusting God and knowing that I can do all things through Christ, strengthening me.

I was at the end of another phase and could step back, smile, and embrace what God did for me. I was beyond blessed; I am a living testimony. The journey, the process, and the cancer diagnosis changed my life. By far, it's the worst thing that has ever happened to me, but in the same breath, I have to admit it is the absolute best thing that has happened to me. I went through emotional pain mental pain, and physical pain after being cut on multiple times due to not getting clear margins and getting medical ports in and out. The anxiety experienced going to the doctor's office, through many machines, facing fears of the unknown. Releasing friendships and the negative voices the enemy tried to put in my head were traumatic. Let's be honest that life doesn't stop so we can heal, so it's important to seek God and renew his strength and mercy daily. The mental and emotional growth that transpired through all the turmoil is priceless; if I had never been diagnosed with cancer, I wouldn't be the woman of God I am today. With that, I challenge you to pause in your personal life and embrace the journey even though you can't wait for this journey to be over. Whether you're a caregiver, a cancer patient, or even just someone reading this book, embrace where you are currently in life, everything you've accomplished thus far, and everything you're about to complete.

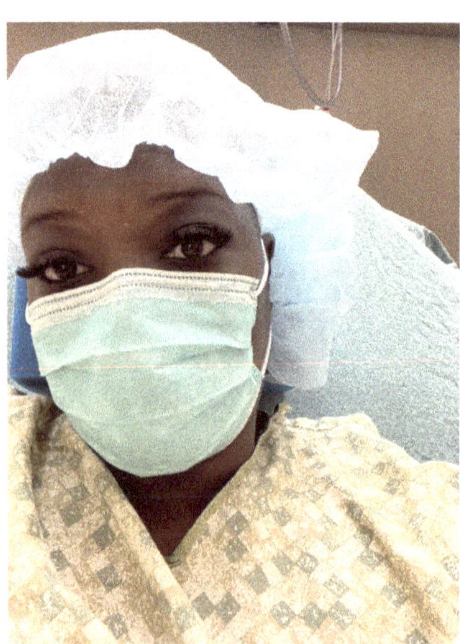
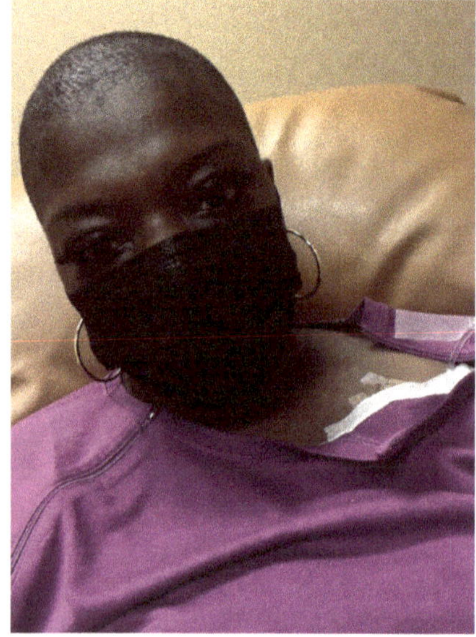

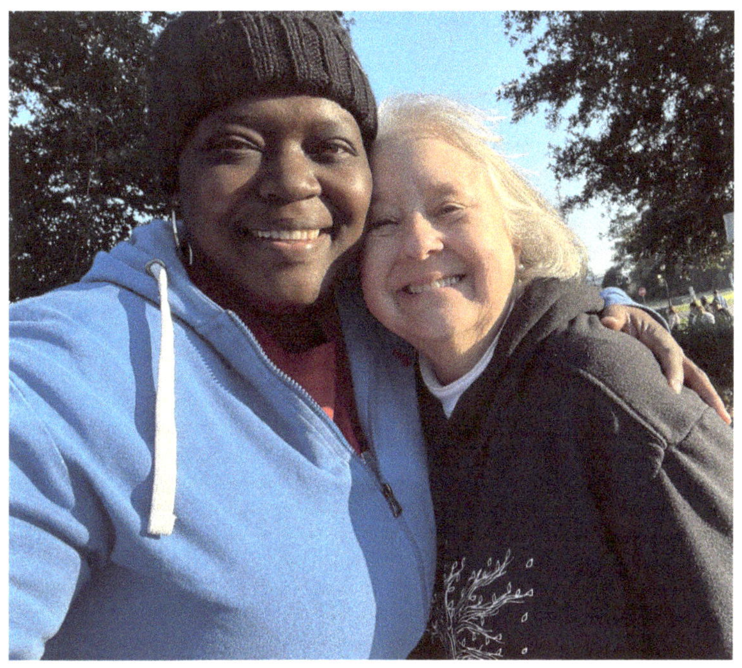

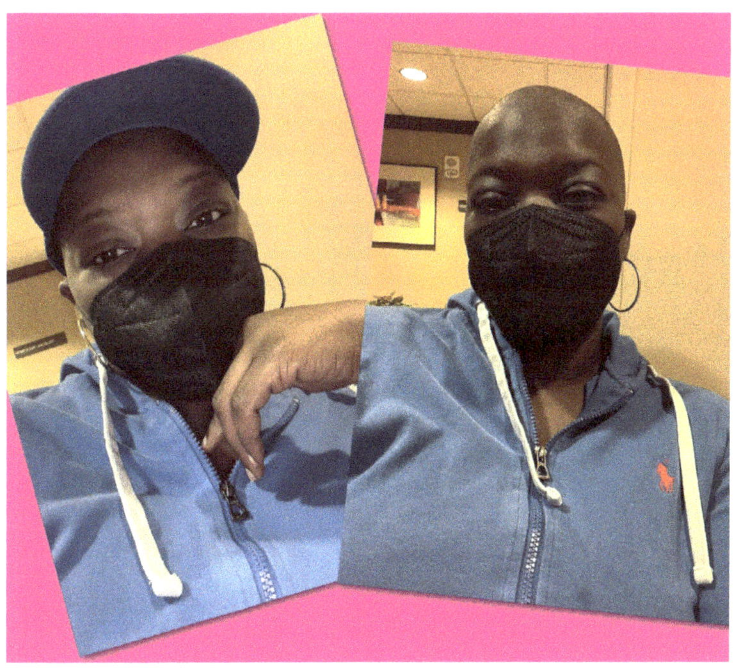

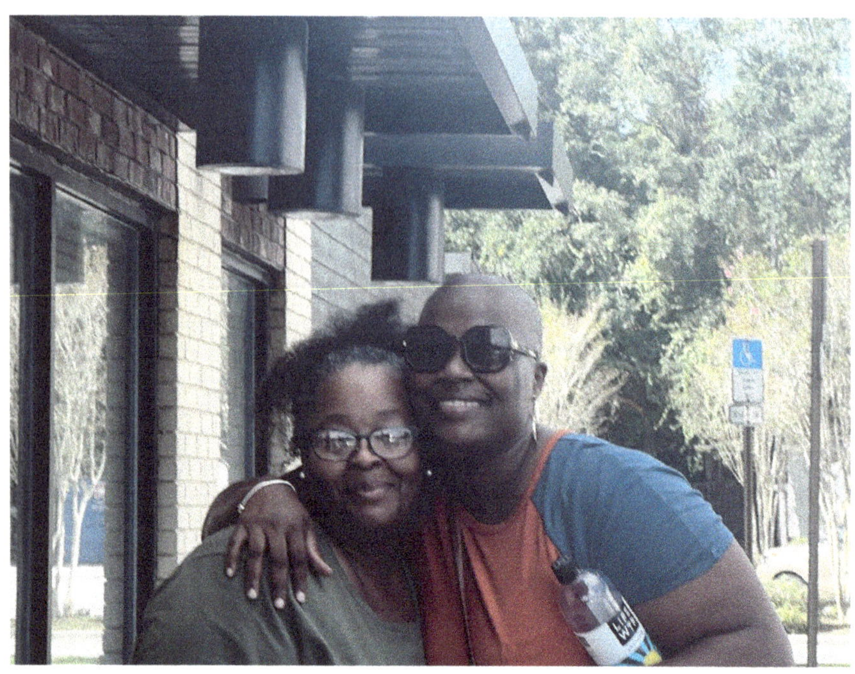

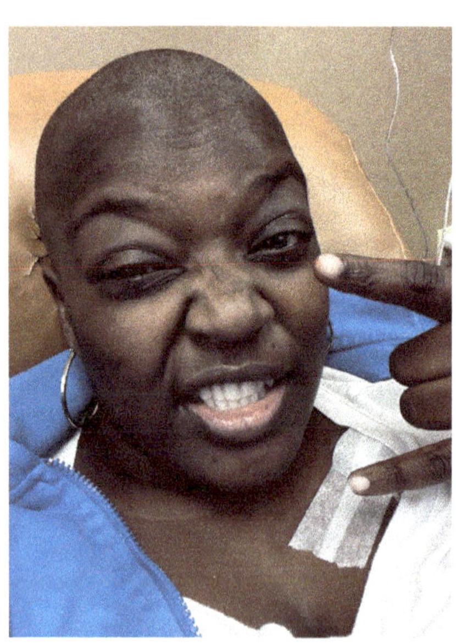

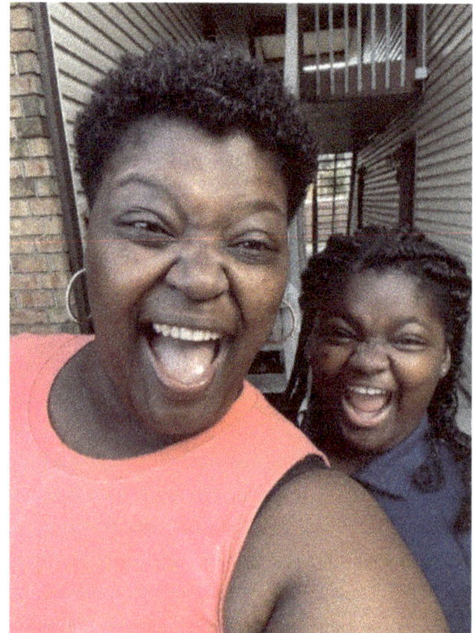

PETALS OF HOPE FROM SURVIVORS AND THRIVERS

During my treatment, I found a quote by Yung Pueblo, that really resonated with me. It goes, "Being OK with not being OK does not make things automatically better, but it does stop you from adding more tension to an already difficult situation." This helped me realize that accepting where I was at that moment was necessary, even if it didn't make everything perfect.
- Melissa Herrmann

Despite being re-diagnosed with metastatic triple-negative breast cancer two years after my first run-in with it, I held my head up high and refused to waver. It's not always easy to keep it together but remember; it takes so much less strength to be positive than to take it as a death sentence.
- Erin Parrish

This journey is a lonely one. No matter what anyone says, this journey is yours alone; others can walk alongside you, but no one can walk for you. The beauty in it all is that you get to choose how you show up for yourself and others in this world. Life will continue to show you the strength you have in you yet challenges you to the core of your being. You are worthy of being here of taking up space for breathing, so breathe life

into the things that light you up, bring a soft smile or tears in the quiet moments, and embrace the you that's come out on the other side. Your light, energy, and soul are needed in this world, and on the days you feel like you want to quit, you can't move forward. Remember that this is your story, your testimony, your moment; live boldly, love well
- Shaina Chafin

Stay happy find the good in each day and keep smiling.
- Tashonna

It's OK to fall apart and it's OK if you don't recognize yourself when you put the pieces back together one of the hardest parts of this journey is rediscovering yourself in the aftermath it's messy and difficult and beautiful and fulfilling don't ever give up on you.
- Staci

It's OK to ask for help with the small daily things you're not a burden to the people who love you and care about you no matter what your brain says
- Rei

This is an experience that separates your „life into three parts part one is your diagnosis and the emotional roller coaster doctor appointments and decisions on treatment that you don't understand best piece

of advice have someone who can take notes in here what the doctors are telling you as the patient you only observe so much because it's so emotional and overwhelming Part 2 is getting through the treatment and this is a very difficult journey for each of us this part is physically emotionally and mentally draining try to find comfort in the little sparks or the times you may feel OK do what you can when you can and allow yourself grace when you just cannot thoughts people will ask you what you need and please take them up on this we all need kindness and to help others when they are in need you or someone you love should make a list and share this with those who want to support this could be picking up a child after school sending lunches or sitting with you at an appointment Part 3 is now what do I do this is the challenging because much as changed yeah life is still moving forward find someone to talk to so that you can figure out how to grieve and deal with all that has happened each day continue to take another step forward to this new normal allow yourself all the feels when they come life slowly finds a new pace and you begin to discover who you are after going through a lot
- Claudia

So much of what others say to you is what keeps them comfortable don't take it too personal anyone who isn't willing to sit with you during these heavy and uncomfortable times they aren't your people.
- Falon